Vegan Slow Cooker

50 Delicious Vegan Recipes to Lose Weight Fast

Introduction

I want to thank you and congratulate you for downloading the book, *"Vegan Slow Cooker: 50 Delicious Vegan Recipes to Lose Weight Fast"*.

This book contains proven steps and strategies on how to prepare delicious and nutritious vegan slow cooker dishes.

You will find a wide variety of flavorful recipes for slow cooker soups, stews, chowders, chilis, main courses, snacks, and even desserts! All of these recipes make use of healthy vegan ingredients that are guaranteed to keep you full with low caloric count.

Thanks again for downloading this book, I hope you enjoy it!

Table of Contents

Chapter 1 - Soups

Carrot and Coconut Curry Bisque

Makes: 2 servings

Ingredients:

- 1/2 onion, diced
- 1 lb baby carrots
- 1 Tbsp grated fresh ginger
- 1/8 tsp cayenne pepper
- 1/2 Tbsp curry powder
- 1/2 fully ripe banana, peeled
- 7 oz canned coconut milk
- 1 lime, juiced
- 1/2 tsp kosher salt
- Optional: fresh flat-leaf parsley, for garnish

Directions:

1. In a 3 quart slow cooker, combine all of the ingredients. Cover and cook for 5 to 6 hours on low, or until onions and carrots soften.

2. With an immersion blender, blend everything until smooth. Garnish with parsley.

Chunky Artichoke Soup

Makes: 2 servings

Ingredients:

- 8 oz fresh button mushrooms, sliced
- 1/2 onion, diced
- 1 cloves garlic, minced
- 8 1/2 oz canned artichoke hearts, undrained
- 1/4 tsp kosher salt
- 1/4 tsp ground black pepper
- 1/8 tsp dried oregano
- 1/8 tsp ground sage
- 1/8 tsp crushed red pepper flakes
- 1/2 cup vegetable broth
- 1/2 cup heavy soy cream

Directions:

1. Place skillet over medium heat and cook onion, garlic, and mushrooms until softened. Transfer into 2 quart slow cooker.

2. Strain artichoke liquids into slow cooker and chop the artichoke hearts before adding them into the mixture. Pour in all the seasonings and the broth. Cover and cook for 4 to 5 hours on low.

3. In a small bowl, whisk the soy cream until fluffy and fold into the soup. Serve.

Cauliflower in French Onion Soup

Makes: 2 servings

Ingredients:

- 2 Tbsp vegan margarine, melted
- 2 yellow onions, sliced into thin rings
- 3 cups vegetable broth
- 1/2 Tbsp sugar
- 1/4 cup dry sherry
- 1/4 tsp kosher salt
- 1/8 tsp ground black pepper
- 1/2 small head cauliflower, cut into florets
- 2 slices vegan Swiss cheese or silken tofu

Directions:

1. In a 2 quart vegan cooker, combine 1 tablespoon melted margarine and onions. Add broth, sherry, salt, pepper, and sugar. Cover and cook for 6 to 7 hours on low or 3 to 4 hours on high, or until onions are completely wilted.

2. Put cauliflower in microwavable dish and microwave for 2 minutes on high or until al dente. Drain liquids and mash. Divide cauliflower into two servings and form into a patty.

3. In a skillet over medium heat, melt 1 tablespoon margarine and cook cauliflower patties until golden brown on both sides.

4. Divide French onion soup between 2 oven-safe bowls and place fried cauliflower patty on top of each. Add vegan cheese or tofu and broil for 1 minute or until cheese melts. Serve.

Roasted Butternut Squash Soup

Makes: 2 to 3 servings

Ingredients:

- 1 large onion
- 1/2 head garlic
- 1 lb butternut squash, seeds removed
- 1 Tbsp olive oil
- 2 cups vegetable broth
- 1/8 cup chopped fresh flat-leaf parsley
- 1/2 Tbsp chopped fresh sage
- 1/4 cup and 2 Tbsp chopped fresh thyme or 1/8 tsp dried thyme
- Salt
- Pepper

Directions:

1. Preheat oven to 375 degrees F.

2. Rub oil on the onion, garlic, and squash. Place, exposed insides facing own on a baking sheet. Bake for 45 minutes or until soft.

3. Spoon flesh from butternut squash and place into 2 quart slow cooker. Remove skins from onion and garlic and add to slow cooker. Add herbs and broth. Cover and cook for 4 hours on low, or until flavors combine.

4. With an immersion blender, blend to a desired consistency. Season with salt and pepper to taste.

Shiitake Mushroom and Tofu Soup

Makes: 2 servings

Ingredients:

- 3 cups vegetable broth
- 6 oz extra firm tofu, cut into small cubes
- 1/2 inch fresh ginger, peeled and grated
- 1/2 Tbsp gluten-free soy sauce
- 1 1/2 green onions, thinly sliced
- 1/4 cup dried shiitake mushrooms, coarsely chopped

Directions:

1. Combine broth, tofu, ginger, and soy sauce in 2 quart slow cooker. Add mushrooms and green onion. Stir and cover.

2. Cook for 4 to 5 hours on low. Mushrooms should swell and absorb the flavor.

Spinach and Tomato Soup

Makes: 2 to 3 servings

Ingredients:

- 1/2 onion, diced
- 1 Tbsp olive oil
- 2 cloves garlic, diced
- 2 stalks celery, thinly sliced
- 13 oz prepared pasta sauce
- 7 oz canned fire-roasted tomatoes, undrained
- 1 cup vegetable broth
- 5 oz spinach
- 1/2 Tbsp dried Italian seasoning
- 1/4 tsp kosher salt
- 1/4 tsp ground black pepper
- 1 cup shredded vegan Swiss cheese

Directions:

1. Heat oil in a skillet over medium heat and saute celery, onion, and garlic until soft.

2. Transfer to 3 quart slow cooker and add tomatoes and sauce, broth, and spinach. Add seasoning, salt, and pepper. Cover and cook for 6 hours on low, stirring to distribute spinach.

3. Divide vegan cheese between serving bowls and add soup over each. Serve.

Tangy Black Bean Soup

Makes: 4 servings

Ingredients:

- 1/2 lb dried black beans, soaked overnight and drained
- 7 oz canned diced tomatoes, drained
- 1/2 red bell pepper, diced
- 1 clove garlic, chopped
- 1/2 tsp of ground: cinnamon, allspice, cumin, chipotle chili
- 1/2 orange, juiced
- 1/2 lime, juiced
- 2 cups vegetable broth
- 1/2 lemon, sliced into 4 wedges

Directions:

1. In a 3 quart slow cooker, combine first 4 ingredients and all ground spices. Add orange and lime juices. Stir well.

2. Cover and cook for 7 hours on low, or until beans are soft. Blend with immersion blender and serve with lemon wedges.

White Bean and Kale Soup

Makes: 4 servings

Ingredients:

- 1/2 lb kale, stems cut off and leaves torn
- 1/2 cup dried white beans, soaked overnight and drained
- 3 cloves garlic, sliced
- 1/2 onion, diced
- 1/2 Tbsp olive oil
- 7 oz canned fire-roasted tomatoes, undrained
- 1/2 tsp kosher salt
- 1/4 tsp crushed red pepper flakes
- 1 1/2 cups vegetable broth
- Optional: grated vegan Parmesan cheese

Directions:

1. In a 3 quart slow cooker, combine the beans, onion, garlic, and kale. Add oil and toss to coat. Add salt, red pepper flakes, tomatoes, and broth. Stir and cover.

2. Cook for 5 to 6 hours on low or for 3 hours on high. Serve with vegan cheese.

Garden Tomato and Spinach Bisque

Makes: 2 to 3 servings

Ingredients:

- 1 lb ripe plum tomatoes, chopped
- 1/2 yellow onion, diced
- 5 oz spinach
- 1/2 cup vegetable broth
- 1/8 cup grated vegan Parmesan
- 1/8 packed dark brown sugar or other sweetener
- 1/2 Tbsp Worcestershire sauce
- 1 tsp dried basil
- 7 oz almond milk

Directions:

1. Pulse vegetables in a blender or food processor. Transfer into 2 quart slow cooker. Add other ingredients, except milk, and cover. Cook for 4 to 5 hours on lo, or for 2 to 3 hours on high.

2. Add almond milk and stir. Cover and cook for 15 minutes on high. Serve.

Curried Eggplant Soup

Makes: 2 servings

Ingredients:

- 1 lb eggplant, peeled and diced
- 7 oz canned diced tomatoes, undrained
- 1/2 onion, diced
- 1/2 tart green apple, peeled and diced
- 1 Tbsp curry powder
- 1/2 Tbsp gluten-free soy sauce
- 1/2 Tbsp maple syrup
- 1/8 tsp kosher salt
- 1/8 tsp cayenne pepper
- 2 cups vegetable broth
- Optional: vegan Feta and/or fresh cilantro leaves, as garnish

Directions:

1. In a 2 quart slow cooker, combine all the ingredients except the garnish. Stir and cover. Cook for 6 to 7 hours on low.

2. With an immersion blender, blend the soup until you get a desired consistency, preferably velvety smooth. Add garnish and serve.

Chapter 2 - Stews

Summer Vegetable Stew

Makes: 4 servings

Ingredients:

- 8 oz frozen red and white pearl onions
- 2 zucchini, cut into 1/4" rounds
- 2 summer squash, washed and cut into 1/4" rounds
- 1/2 cup chopped baby carrots
- 1/4 cup sliced celery
- 1/6 cup dried chickpeas, rinsed
- 2 cups vegetable broth
- 1/2 cup tomato-based pasta sauce
- 1/2 cup water
- 1/2 Tbsp dried Italian seasoning
- 1/4 cup gluten-free penne
- Optional: grated vegan Parmesan

Directions:

1. In a 3 quart slow cooker, combine the first 6 ingredients, then add the broth, sauce, and water. Add seasoning and stir. Cover and cook for 6 hours on low, or until beans become tender.

2. Add pasta and stir. Increase heat to high and cook for 20 minutes. Serve with vegan Parmesan.

Super Skinny Vegetable Stew

Makes: 4 servings

Ingredients:

- 2 1/2 cups vegetable broth
- 1/2 onion, diced
- 1 carrot, diced
- 1/4 lb frozen green beans
- 1/4 head cabbage, chopped
- 2 cloves garlic, minced
- 1 Tbsp tomato paste
- 1/2 tsp each of dried: basil, oregano
- 1/2 tsp kosher salt
- 1/4 tsp ground black pepper
- 1 small zucchini, diced
- Optional: grated vegan Parmesan cheese

Directions:

1. In a 3 quart slow cooker, combine all ingredients, except zucchini and cheese, and stir.

2. Cover and cook for 6 to 7 hours on low, or until onion becomes soft. Add zucchini 1 hour before end of cooking time. Add cheese over each serving, if preferred.

Tofu and Grape Stew

Makes: 2 servings

Ingredients:

- 1 1/2 cups cubed tofu
- 1/2 cup thinly sliced carrots
- 1 cup seedless grapes, quartered
- 1/4 cup each: red wine, water
- 1 bouillon cube
- 1 tsp dried tarragon
- 1/4 cup minced fresh parsley
- Salt and Pepper
- 1 cup cooked whole wheat couscous

Directions:

1. Combine all ingredients, except parsley, salt, pepper, and couscous. Cook for 8 hours on low.

2. Stir in parsley, salt, and pepper before serving over couscous.

Green and Black Bean Stew with Tofu

Makes: 2 servings

Ingredients:

- 3 cups green beans, cut 1/2" thick
- 1/4 cup water
- 7 1/2 oz firm tofu, cut into small cubes
- 2 Tbsp black bean paste
- 1 Tbsp white vinegar
- 2 tsp sesame oil
- 1/4 tsp chili garlic paste
- Cooked brown rice, for serving

Directions:

1. Combine green beans and water in slow cooker. Cook for 30 minutes on high.

2. In a bowl, combine tofu, black bean paste, vinegar, oil, and garlic paste.

3. Add tofu mixture to cooked beans and stir well. Cook for 1 hour on high. Serve over rice.

Three Sisters Stew

Makes: 2 servings

Ingredients:

- 1 cup water
- 2/3 cup dry scarlet runner beans, uncooked
- 1 1/2 cups corn
- 1 1/4 tsp cumin
- 3/4 tsp chili powder
- 1 cup summer squash, diced
- 1/2 cup diced tomatoes
- Salt
- Pepper

Directions:

1. Combine first 4 ingredients in slow cooker and cook for 7 hours on low.

2. Increase heat to high and add the rest of the ingredients. Stir well. Cook for 30 minutes or until squash is tender. Serve with gluten-free bread.

Veggie Garden Stew

Makes: 2 servings

Ingredients:

- 1 cup vegetable broth
- 8 oz each: cauliflower florets, sliced mushrooms, cubed potatoes
- 1 medium onion, cut into wedges
- 1 medium tomato, cut into wedges
- 1 clove garlic, minced
- 1/2 bay leaf
- 1/2 tsp dried savory leaves
- 1 small zucchini, sliced
- Salt and pepper
- 1 1/2 cups cooked couscous, warm

Directions:

1. Combine all ingredients, except zucchini, salt, pepper, and couscous, in slow cooker.

2. Cover and cook for 6 hours on low. Add zucchini in the last half hour. Remove bay leaf and serve over couscous.

Chilean Black Bean Stew

Makes: 3 servings

Ingredients:

- 7 1/2 oz canned black beans, drained and rinsed
- 8 oz corn
- 1 medium onion, diced
- 1 small butternut squash, peeled, seeded, and cubed
- 1/8 cup tightly packed chopped basil leaves
- 1/8 tsp cayenne pepper
- 1/4 tsp kosher salt
- 2 cups vegetable broth

Directions:

1. Combine all ingredients in a 3 quart slow cooker and stir to mix.

2. Cover and cook for 4 to 5 hours on low, or until onion becomes translucent.

Sweet and Sour Squash and Potato Stew

Makes: 3 servings

Ingredients:

- 7 1/2 oz canned diced tomatoes, undrained
- 1/2 cup apple juice
- 1 1/2 cups each: peeled and cubed Idaho potatoes, acorn or butternut squash
- 1 cup each: peeled and cubed tart green apples, sweet potatoes
- 3/4 cup corn kernels
- 1/4 cup each: chopped red bell pepper, shallots
- 1 clove garlic, minced
- 3/4 Tbsp each: cider vinegar, maple syrup
- 1/2 bay leaf
- 1/8 tsp ground nutmeg
- 1/8 cup cold water
- 1 Tbsp cornstarch
- Salt and Pepper
- 2 cups cooked jasmine rice, warm

Directions:

1. In a 3 quart slow cooker, mix together all ingredients, except rice, salt, pepper, water, and cornstarch. Cover and cook for 6 hours on low.

2. Increase heat to high and cook for 10 minutes. Mix together water and cornstarch and stir into the stew. Remove bay leaf. Add salt and pepper. Serve over rice.

Lentil Stew with Spiced Couscous

Makes: 3 servings

Ingredients:

- 7 1/2 oz canned diced tomatoes, undrained
- 1 1/2 cups vegetable broth
- 1 cup dried lentils
- 1/2 cup each: chopped red or green bell pepper, onion, carrots, celery
- 1/2 tsp each: dried oregano, minced garlic
- 1/4 tsp ground turmeric
- Salt and Pepper

For Spiced Couscous:

- 1/6 cup sliced green onions
- 1/2 clove garlic, minced
- 1/8 tsp crushed red pepper
- 1/4 tsp ground turmeric
- 1/2 tsp olive oil
- 3/4 cup vegetable broth
- 1/2 cup couscous

Directions:

1. Combine tomatoes, broth, lentils, bell pepper, onion, carrots, celery, garlic, turmeric, and oregano in 3 quart slow cooker. Cover and cook for 6 hours on low. Season with salt and pepper.

2. To make the Spiced couscous, saute green onions, red pepper, turmeric, and garlic in skillet over medium heat until tender. Add broth and bring to a boil. Add couscous. Remove

from heat and set aside, covered, for 5 minutes or until couscous absorbs broth.

3. Serve stew over spiced couscous.

Tofu and Vegetable Stew

Makes: 2 servings

Ingredients:

- 2 cups vegetable broth
- 1 cup each: sliced carrots, red potatoes
- 1/4 cup each: sliced celery, onion
- 5 1/2 oz firm light tofu, cut into 1/2" cubes
- 2 cloves garlic, minced
- 1/2 bay leaf
- 1/2 tsp ground cumin
- 1/4 tsp dried thyme
- 5 oz chopped spinach
- Salt and Pepper

Directions:

1. Combine all ingredients, except salt, pepper, parsley, and spinach, in slow cooker.

2. Cover and cook for 3 hours on high. Add spinach within last 20 minutes of cooking time. Remove bay leaf and season to taste with salt and pepper.

Chapter 3 - Chilis and Chowders

Roasted Garlic and Potato Chowder

Makes: 3 servings

Ingredients:
- 4 baking potatoes, peeled and cubed
- 1 onion, diced
- 2 stalks celery, diced
- 1/2 cup chopped baby carrots
- 1/2 head garlic, peeled
- 1/2 tsp kosher salt
- 1/ tsp ground black pepper
- 2 1/2 cups vegetable broth
- 1/2 cup heavy soy cream

Directions:

1. Combine vegetables in 3 quart slow cooker and season with salt and pepper. Add broth and stir. Cover and cook for 5 to 6 hours on low or until garlic can be mashed.

2. With a potato masher, mash some of the potato cubes to thicken. Add soy cream and stir. Cover and cook for 15 minutes on high or until soup is hot.

Sweet Corn Chowder

Makes: 3 servings

Ingredients:
- 8 oz frozen white corn
- 2 cups vegetable broth
- 1 Yukon Gold potato, peeled and diced
- 2 cloves garlic, minced
- 1/2 tsp kosher salt
- 1/4 tsp ground black pepper
- 1/2 cup heavy soy cream

Directions:

1. Combine all ingredients except cream in a 2 quart slow cooker. Cover and cook for 6 hours on low or until potatoes are bite-tender.

2. With an immersion blender, blend soup to a desired consistency. Stir in soy cream, cover, and cook for 25 minutes on high. Serve hot.

Avocado and Tomato Chowder

Makes: 2 servings

Ingredients:

- 1 cup vegetable broth
- 1 1/2 cups peeled and cubed potatoes
- 4 oz vegan "turkey" breast, cubed
- 1/2 cup corn kernels
- 1/2 cup chopped plum potatoes
- 1/2 tsp dried thyme
- 1/2 cup cubed avocado
- 1/2 lime, juiced
- 2 slices veggie bacon, cooked and crumbled
- Salt and pepper

Directions:

1. Combine first 6 ingredients in 3 quart slow cooker. Cover and cook for 4 hours on high. Add the rest of the ingredients and stir.

Sweet Onion and Bean Chowder

Makes: 4 servings

Ingredients:

- 2 cups vegetable broth
- 7 1/ oz Great Northern beans, rinsed and drained
- 3/4 lb onions, thinly sliced
- 1/3 tsp dried thyme leaves
- Salt and pepper
- Garlic croutons, for serving

Directions:

1. Combine all ingredients except salt, pepper, and croutons, in 3 quart slow cooker. Cover and cook for 4 hours on high. Season with salt and pepper. Serve with garlic croutons.

Corn and Potato Chowder

Makes: 2 servings

Ingredients:

- 1 cup each: vegetable broth, cubed potatoes
- 1 small onion, chopped
- 1 cup corn kernels
- 1/4 cup sliced celery
- 1/2 tsp dried thyme
- 1 cup almond milk, divided
- 1 Tbsp cornstarch
- Salt and Pepper

Directions:

1. Combine all ingredients, except milk, cornstarch, salt and pepper, in 3 quart slow cooker. Cover and cook for 3 to 4 hours on high. Add 1/2 cup milk within last half hour of cooking time.

2. Combine 1/2 cup milk and cornstarch and stir into chowder. Season with salt and pepper.

Indian-spiced Chili

Makes: 3 servings

Ingredients:

- 7 1/2 oz canned kidney beans, drained and rinsed
- 7 1/2 oz canned chickpeas, drained and rinsed
- 7 oz canned diced tomatoes, undrained
- 1 lb red potatoes, washed and cubed
- 1/2 onion diced
- 2 stalks celery, diced
- 1 1/2 Tbsp curry powder
- 1/2 Tbsp chili powder
- 1/2 tsp ground turmeric
- 1/4 tsp garam masala
- 1/2 tsp kosher salt
- 2 cups vegetable broth
- 1 jalapeno pepper
- Corn tortillas, for serving

Directions:

1. In a 3 quart slow cooker, combine all ingredients except corn tortillas and jalapenos. Add jalapenos on top, uncrushed.

2. Cover and cook for 6 hours on low, or until potatoes become tender and onions become translucent. Remove jalapenos. Serve with corn tortilla wedges.

Black Bean Chili

Makes: 3 servings

Ingredients:

- 15 oz canned black beans, undrained
- 14 oz canned crushed tomatoes, undrained
- 7 1/2 canned white corn, undrained
- 1/8 cup dried minced onion
- 1/2 Tbsp unsweetened cocoa powder
- 1 Tbsp chili powder
- 1/2 tsp each: ground cumin, garlic powder
- Toppings: vegan Cheddar cheese, soy cream

Directions:

1. In a 3 quart slow cooker, combine all the ingredients, except the toppings, and stir well. Cover and cook for 4 to 5 hours on low.

2. Take out half a cup of the chili and blend with an immersion blender, then return to the pot and stir. Top with cheese or cream, if preferred.

Lentil and Corn Chili

Makes: 4 servings

Ingredients:

- 14 oz canned diced tomatoes, undrained
- 8 oz dried green or brown lentils, rinsed
- 1/2 onion, diced
- 1/2 cup chopped celery
- 2 cloves garlic, minced
- 1/8 cup chopped fresh cilantro leaves
- 8 oz frozen white corn, thawed
- 1 Tbsp chili powder
- 1 Tbsp ground cumin
- 1/ tsp kosher salt
- 1/4 tsp cayenne pepper
- 1 cup vegetable broth

Directions:

1. Combine all ingredients in a 3 quart slow cooker and stir to combine.

2. Cover and cook for 6 hours on low. Stir before you serve.

Chocolate Chili

Makes: 3 servings

Ingredients:

- 1/2 lb dried small red beans
- 1/2 cup diced baby carrots
- 1/2 yellow onion, diced
- 2 cloves garlic, chopped
- 1/2 Tbsp sugar
- 1 1/2 Tbsp chili powder
- 1/4 Tbsp ground chipotle chili
- 1/2 tsp of each: paprika, dried oregano, ground cumin, kosher salt
- 14 oz canned crushed tomatoes
- 1/4 cup brewed coffee
- 1/4 cup water
- 1/2 oz unsweetened baking chocolate

Directions:

1. Put beans in a pot and cover with water. Cover and boil for 6 to 8 minutes on medium-high heat. Set beans aside in the hot water for an hour to remove toxins; keep covered. Drain and pour beans into slow cooker.

2. Add the rest of the ingredients into the slow cooker. Stir well. Cover and cook for 7 hours on low, or until beans become soft. Stir before you serve.

Barbecue Bean Chili

Makes: 4 servings

Ingredients:

- 1/2 lb crumbled tempeh
- 1/2 lb dried small red beans
- 1 onion, diced
- 2 ripe tomatoes, chopped
- 3 cloves garlic, chopped
- 1/2 cup frozen white corn
- 1/2 cup gluten-free, vegan barbecue sauce
- 1/8 cup minced fresh cilantro leaves
- 1 Tbsp chili powder
- 1/2 Tbsp ground cumin
- 1/2 cup vegetable broth

Directions:

1. Pour beans in a pot and cover with water. Cook for 10 minutes to a boil. Set aside in hot water for 1 hour to remove potential toxins, then drain and pour into 3 quart slow cooker.

2. Saute onion, garlic, and tempeh in a lightly greased skillet over medium heat. Pour into slow cooker and add the rest of the ingredients. Stir and cover.

3. Cook for 6 to 7 hours on low, or until beans become split and are fork-tender.

Chapter 4 - Main Course

Cheesy Lentil Bake

Makes: 3 to 4 servings

Ingredients:

- 7 oz canned diced tomatoes, undrained
- 1 cup dried brown or green lentils, rinsed
- 1/4 cup chopped baby carrots
- 1/2 red onion, diced
- 1/4 cup sliced celery
- 1/2 Tbsp herbes de Provence
- 1/4 tsp kosher salt
- 1/8 tsp ground black pepper
- 1 1/4 cups vegetable broth
- 1 cup vegan Cheddar, shredded
- 1/2 cup vegan Mozzarella, shredded

Directions:

1. Combine all ingredients, except the vegan cheeses, in a 2 quart slow cooker. Top with the vegan cheeses.

2. Cover and cook for 4 hours on low, or until cheeses are completely melted and lentils become al dente.

Barbecue Beans

Makes: 3 to 4 servings

Ingredients:

- 1/2 lb crumbled tempeh
- 1/2 onion, diced
- 2 cloves garlic, minced
- 15 oz canned navy beans, drained and rinsed
- 14 oz canned baked beans
- 1/2 cup gluten-free vegan barbecue sauce
- 1 Tbsp Worcestershire sauce
- 1/8 cup yellow mustard
- 1/4 tsp each: kosher salt, ground black pepper
- 2 slices veggie bacon
- Cornbread, for serving

Directions:

1. Cook onion, garlic, and crumbled tempeh in a lightly greased skillet over medium heat until browned. Transfer mixture into slow cooker and add beans. Add the sauces, mustard, salt, and pepper. Place veggie bacon on top.

2. Cover and cook for 6 hours on low, or on high for 2 to 3 hours. Serve with cornbread.

Tomato Curried Lentils

Makes: 2 servings

Ingredients:

- 1/2 cup dried green or brown lentils, rinsed
- 1 cup vegetable broth
- 7 oz canned diced tomatoes, undrained
- 2 cloves garlic, diced
- 1/2 onion, diced
- 1 tsp curry powder
- 1/4 tsp ground black pepper
- Hot cooked brown rice, for serving

Directions:

1. Combine all ingredients, except brown rice, in 2 quart slow cooker. Cover and cook for 4 hours on low. Serve with brown rice.

Carrot Risotto

Makes: 1 to 2 servings

Ingredients:

- 1/2 Tbsp melted margarine
- 3/4 cups Arborio rice
- 1/4 onion, finely diced
- 1/2 cup shredded carrots
- 2 cloves garlic, minced
- 1/4 tsp each: kosher salt, ground black pepper
- 1 1/2 cups vegetable broth
- 1/2 cup dry white wine
- 1/2 cup vegan Parmesan

Directions:

1. Grease slow cooker with margarine, the add rice and stir to coat. Add the rest of the ingredients, except vegan Parmesan.

2. Cover and cook for 2 hours on high, or until rice is tender. Stir vegan Parmesan in. Let sit, uncovered, for 8 minutes before you serve.

Eggplant Steaks with Baked Garlic

Makes: 2 servings

Ingredients:

- 1 medium eggplant, cut into 6 slices
- 1 Tbsp olive oil
- 1/2 tsp paprika
- 1/2 head garlic, crushed
- 1/8 cup torn fresh basil leaves
- 3 oz vegan mozzarella, sliced
- 7 oz canned fire-roasted tomatoes, undrained

Directions:

1. Grease 3 quart slow cooker with 1/2 tablespoon olive oil and layer eggplant slices on top. Brush remaining oil on top of eggplants. Add paprika, garlic, basil, cheese, and tomatoes.

2. Cover and cook for 3 hours on low or until cheese melts and eggplant is tender.

Mushroom and Bean Ragout

Makes: 3 servings

Ingredients:

- 1/2 lb fresh cremini mushrooms, sliced thinly
- 2 cloves garlic, minced
- 1 onion, chopped
- 1/2 Tbsp chopped fresh or 3/4 tsp dried thyme
- 1/4 tsp each: kosher salt, ground pepper
- 1/2 Tbsp olive oil
- 14 oz canned diced tomatoes, undrained
- 7 1/2 oz canned cannellini beans, drained and rinsed
- Hot cooked polenta, for serving

Directions:

1. In a 3 quart slow cooker, put mushrooms on bottom an add the rest of the ingredients on top. Stir to coat in oil and cover.

2. Cook for 6 to 7 hours on low or until tomatoes and mushrooms have broken down. Serve over polenta.

Saffron Risotto

Makes: 1 serving

Ingredients:

- 1/2 Tbsp margarine, melted
- 1 1/2 Tbsp olive oil
- 3/4 cup Arborio rice
- 1/2 tsp dried minced onion
- 1/8 tsp ground black pepper
- 1/2 tsp saffron threads
- 2 cups vegetable broth
- 1/4 cup vegan Parmesan, grated
- 1/8 cup dry white wine

Directions:

1. In a 2 quart slow cooker, combine margarine and oil. Stir rice in it and add the rest of the ingredients. Stir to combine. Cover and cook for 2 to 3 hours on high. Stir before you serve.

Vegan Tacos

Makes: 3 servings

Ingredients:

- 1 cup dried green or brown lentils, rinsed
- 1 cup vegetable broth
- 1/2 onion, diced
- 1/2 oz packet taco seasoning
- Taco shells, for serving
- For toppings: vegan Cheddar, avocado slices, soy cream, black olives, salsa

Directions:

1. In a 2 quart slow cooker, combine lentils, broth, onion, and taco seasoning.

2. Cover and cook for 4 hours on low, or until lentils become al dente. Serve in taco shells with toppings.

Mediterranean Eggplant

Makes: 2 servings

Ingredients:

- 1/2 Tbsp olive oil
- 1/2 lb eggplant, peeled and cut into 1" cubes
- 1/2 onion, thinly sliced
- 1/2 red bell pepper, seeded and thinly sliced
- 2 ripe tomatoes, diced
- 2 cloves garlic, chopped
- 1/2 small zucchini, thinly sliced
- 1 tsp dried basil
- 2 oz vegan tofu feta

Directions:

1. Combine all ingredients, except vegan feta, in 3 quart slow cooker. Toss to combine well.

2. Cover and cook for 4 hours on low or for 1 1/2 hours on high. Add crumbled tofu feta on top.

Maple Beans and Spinach Dinner

Makes: 2 to 3 servings

Ingredients:

- 7 1/2 oz canned chickpeas, drained and rinsed
- 7 1/2 oz canned black beans, drained and rinsed
- 1/2 onion, finely diced
- 1 medium sweet potato, peeled and chopped
- 2 cloves garlic, minced
- 1 tsp ground cumin
- 1/4 tsp each: ground coriander, kosher salt, ground black pepper
- 1/8 cup maple syrup
- 1/2 lemon, juiced
- 6 oz fresh baby spinach
- Hot cooked brown basmati rice, for serving

Directions:

1. In a 3 quart slow cooker, combine all ingredients, except spinach and rice, and stir to coat the vegetables and beans. Add the spinach on top.

2. Cover and cook for 3 hours on low or for 2 hours on high. Stir before serving with rice.

Chapter 5 - Snacks and Desserts

Pumpkin Caramel Barley

Makes: 4 servings

Ingredients:

- 1 cup barley
- 4 cups unsweetened almond milk
- 8 Tbsp coconut caramel sauce
- For Coconut Caramel Sauce:
- 28 oz full fat coconut milk
- 2 cups packed brown sugar
- 2 cups pumpkin puree
- 1 tsp ground cinnamon
- 1/4 tsp ground cardamom
- 1/4 tsp ground allspice
- A pinch of cloves

Directions:

1. Make the coconut caramel sauce by combining the ingredients in the slow cooker. Cook for 9 hours on low. Transfer into a sterilized glass jar and store in the refrigerator.

2. Combine barley and almond milk in the slow cooker. Cook for 9 hours on low.

3. Stir barley and add coconut caramel sauce.

Bananas Foster

Makes: 4 servings

Ingredients:
- 1 cup and 6 Tbsp almond milk
- 4 medium bananas, mashed
- 2 tsp rum flavoring
- 2 Tbsp ground flaxseeds mixed with 4 Tbsp water
- 1 tsp ground cinnamon
- 5 cups old gluten-free bread, cut into chunks
- Maple syrup, for serving

Directions:

1. Combine milk, rum, flax mixture, cinnamon, stevia, and bananas in a bowl. Add bread and set aside for 15 minutes to absorb.

2. Line slow cooker with parchment paper. Transfer mixture into it and cook for 9 hours on low.

Soy Noshers

Makes: 4 servings

Ingredients:

- 3/4 cup roasted soy beans
- 1/2 cup dried blueberries or cranberries
- 1/4 cup each: mini pretzel twists, wheat squares cereal
- 1/3 tsp each: crushed dried thyme, dried rosemary
- Garlic salt
- Vegetable cooking spray

Directions:

1. Set slow cooker on high and heat for 15 minutes. Combine berries, soy beans, pretzels, and cereal. Spray with vegetable oil and toss. Sprinkle herbs and toss.

2. Cover and cook for 2 hours on low. Stir every 20 minutes. Increase heat to high and cook, uncovered, for 20 minutes. Stir occasionally. Season with garlic salt.

Spinach and Artichoke Dip

Makes: 1o servings

Ingredients:

- 8 oz artichoke hearts, drained and finely chopped
- 1/2 cup each: vegan Parmesan, soy cream
- 1 tsp lemon juice
- 1/2 green onion, thinly sliced
- 1 tsp minced garlic
- Salt
- Cayenne pepper
- 1/2 cup chopped spinach
- 1/4 cup chopped roasted red pepper
- Dippers: assorted vegetables, bread sticks

Directions:

1. Combine all ingredients, except salt, cayenne pepper, and dippers. in a 1 1/2 quart slow cooker. Cover and cook for 1 hour until hot.

2. Season with salt and cayenne pepper to taste. Serve with dippers.

Toasted Onion Dip

Makes: 12 servings

Ingredients:

- 4 Tbsp dried onion flakes
- 1/2 lb soy cream cheese
- 1/2 cup nut cream or butter
- 2 small green onions, chopped
- 1 clove garlic, minced
- 1/2 cup almond milk
- 1 tsp lemon juice
- 3 drops red pepper sauce
- Salt and White Pepper
- Dippers: assorted vegetables, bread sticks

Directions:

1. Saute onion flakes in skillet over medium-low heat until toasted. Transfer into 1 1/2 quart slow cooker and add the rest of the ingredients, except lemon juice, pepper, sauce, salt, and pepper.

2. Cover and cook for 1 hour or until hot. Add lemon juice, red pepper sauce, and season with salt and white pepper. Serve with dippers.

Apple and Cranberry Compote

Makes: 3 servings

Ingredients:

- 1/4 cup dried cranberries
- 2 cups peeled, cored, and sliced apples
- 1/6 cup packed light brown sugar or other sweetener
- 1/2 tsp ground cinnamon
- 1/8 tsp each: salt, ground nutmeg
- 1/3 cup granola with nuts

Directions:

1. Mix together all ingredients, except granola, in a 2 quart slow cooker. Cover and cook for 1 1/2 hours on high or until apples become tender.

2. Serve with granola sprinkled on top.

Fast and Easy Brownies

Makes: 8 servings

Ingredients:

- 10 oz vegan brownie mix
- 2 Tbsp melted margarine
- 1/2 cup chopped walnuts

Directions:

1. Prepare brownie mix based on manufacturer's instructions. Add margarine and walnuts.

2. Pour batter into a greased spring-form pan and put it on the rack of a 3 quart slow cooker. Cover and cook for 5 hours or until done. To check, poke the center of the brownie with a toothpick; if it comes out almost clean it is ready.

3. Cool on a wire rack, then cut into squares.

Apple Chocolate Chip Pudding

Makes: 2 servings

Ingredients:

- 2 cups old whole wheat bread
- 1 cup almond milk
- 1 1/2 cups peeled minced apple
- 1 Tbsp ground flaxseeds combined with 2 Tbsp warm water
- 1/3 cup chopped nuts
- 1/4 cup sugar
- 1/4 cup minced vegan chocolate chips

Directions:

1. Line slow cooker with parchment paper.

2. In a mixing bowl, soak bread with apples in milk, sugar and flaxseed mixture for 10 minutes. Transfer into slow cooker. Add chocolate and nuts. Cook for 1 1/2 hours on high.

Blueberry Lemon Cake

Makes: 2 servings

Ingredients:

- 1/4 tsp stevia plus 1 tsp agave nectar
- 1/2 cup whole wheat pastry flour
- 1/4 tsp baking powder
- 1/3 cup unsweetened almond milk
- 1 tsp ground flaxseeds combined with 2 tsp warm water
- 1/4 cup blueberries
- 1 tsp olive oil
- 1/2 tsp lemon zest
- 1/4 tsp each: lemon and vanilla extracts

Directions:

1. Line slow cooker with parchment paper.

2. Combine dry ingredients in a bowl. Combine wet ingredients in another bowl.

3. Combine dry and wet mixtures well and pour into slow cooker. Spread evenly. Place a paper towel between the lid and the pot. Cook for 1 hour on high.

Spiced Apple Crumble

Makes: 2 servings

Ingredients:

- 2 cups chopped apple
- 1/8 cup packed brown sugar
- 1/4 cup pecans, minced
- 1/8 tsp each: ground ginger, nutmeg
- 1/4 tsp each: ground cinnamon, cardamom
- Allspice and cloves

For topping:

- 1/4 cup rolled oats
- 1/8 cup packed brown sugar
- 1/8 cup whole-wheat pastry flour
- 1 Tbsp almond milk
- 1/8 tsp each: ground cinnamon, cardamom
- 1/16 tsp each: ground ginger, nutmeg
- Allspice and cloves

Directions:

1. Combine first 6 ingredients in slow cooker.

2. In a mixing bowl, combine topping ingredients and drop gradually over filling using teaspoon.

3. Cook for 1 hour on high. Serve with soy ice cream if preferred.

Conclusion

Thank you again for downloading this book!

I hope this book was able to help you to lose weight by sticking to an all-vegan diet with the help of this book.

The next step is to create an effective diet and exercise plan that will help you lose weight and keep it at a healthy fitness level.

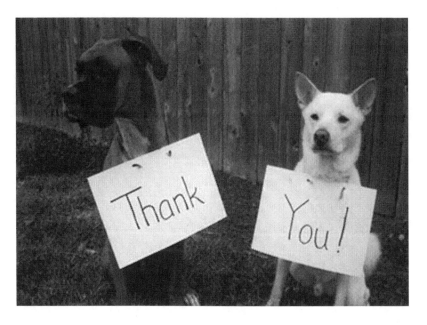

Finally, if you enjoyed this book, then I'd like to ask you for a favor, would you be kind enough to leave a review for this book on Amazon? It'd be greatly appreciated!

Thank you and good luck!

Made in the USA
San Bernardino, CA
29 September 2017